DASH DIET
COOKBOOK FOR TWO

50 SIMPLE, TASTY RECIPES FOR BEGINNERS. DISCOVER A COMPLETE GUIDE ON WHAT KIND OF FOOD IS BETTER TO AVOID FOLLOWING THE LOW SODIUM DASH DIET. IF YOU OR YOUR LOVED ONE ARE DIAGNOSED WITH HYPERTENSION, ACT NOW AND START WITH THE DASH DIET.

TABLE OF CONTENTS

CHAPTER 1

INTRODUCTION

The Dash Diet Cookbook will have you hacking out your cutlery in no time so you can finally become a healthier human being! It's all about being healthy and learning to enjoy the foods you eat again. We have concluded that Dash Diet Cookbook is an excellent way of losing weight and following a healthy, balanced diet. The Dash Diet Cookbook is a collection of simple recipes that are easy to prepare and incredibly tasty. Many different styles of cooking are featured, so you can find something that works for you. The Dash Diet Cookbook is perfect for anyone who wants to eat better and feel great while saving money and time.

The DASH diet's primary focus is on grains, vegetables, and fruits because these foods are higher fiber foods and will make you feel full longer. Consume whole grains six to eight times daily, vegetables four to six servings daily, and fruit four to five servings daily. In addition, low-fat dairy is an essential part of the diet and should be eaten two to three times daily. And there should be six or fewer servings daily of fish, poultry, and lean meat.

A DASH diet can be easily integrated into daily life simply because it uses foods that are available in conventional grocery stores. Then, depending on your calorie requirement, the amounts consumed of the individual foods result.

WHAT CAN I EAT?

Allowed foods are:
>   plenty of fresh vegetables, especially lots of greens - almost without restriction
>   Fresh fruit
>   lean meats, especially white meat (chicken, turkey)
>   Whole grain / whole grain products
>   fish
>   Protein-rich foods
>   Foods with unsaturated and healthy fats such as nuts and avocados
>   Healthy oils with an optimal Omega3 / 6 ratio such as olive oil and coconut oil
>   Lean dairy products
>   Nuts, seeds, legumes

In small amounts:
>   alcohol
>   coffee
>   animal fats, especially red meat
>   Sweets and sugar

Avoid as much as possible:
>   Ready meals and canned food
>   Sausages
>   Bakery products
>   hydrogenated vegetable fats such as palm fat
>   Sunflower oil (poor omega3 / 6 ratio)
>   pickled and smoked foods

How DASH Diet Help You Lose Weight And Lower Blood Pressure
Despite not being specifically designed for weight loss, the Dash Diet does indeed help to trim down your weight through various indirect means.

While the DASH diet does not include stress reductions in calories, it influences you to fill up your diet with very nutrient-dense food instead of calorie-rich food, which quickly helps to shed a few pounds!

Since you will be on a heavy diet of veggies and fruits, you will be consuming lots of fiber, which is also believed to help weight loss.

Aside from that, the diet also helps to control your appetite since cleaner, and nutrient-dense foods will keep you satisfied throughout the day! In addition, lower food intake will further contribute to weight loss.

And while you are at it, the program will indirectly encourage you to carry out a daily workout to keep your body healthy and fit. Therefore, following the DASH Diet program while working out will significantly enhance the effectiveness of the program.

Understanding the food groups

To keep things simple, let me break down the food groups to understand the food regime of the program better.

Eat as much as you want

Grains, such as barley, wheat bread, wheat pasta, etc.

Meats, such as eggs, lean beef, lean chicken, lean pork

Seafood, such as fish, Shrimp, and Salmon

Fruits such as apples, bananas, cherries, grapes, blackberries, mangoes, etc.

Vegetables such as artichokes, broccoli, Brussels sprouts, carrots, bell peppers, green beans, etc.

Limit Your Servings

Healthy vegetable oils, such as canola, corn, olive, etc.

Condiments

Dairy such as Greek yogurt, skim milk, low-fat milk, low-fat cheese

Nuts, legumes, and seeds such as almonds, cashews, flax seeds, hazelnuts, lentils, pecans, kidney beans

Red meats

Eat Rarely

Sweets such as beverages, jams, jellies, sugars, sweet yogurt

Saturated fats such as bacon, cholesterol, coconuts, fatty meats

Sodium-rich foods such as canned fruits, canned vegetables, gravy pizza, etc.

Understanding daily proportions

Controlling your daily portions is crucial when it comes to the Dash Diet program. While the critical component here is to keep your sodium intake at a low level, there are other things that you must consider.

So, to properly maintain your DASH diet, you should:

Consume more fruits, low-fat dairy foods, and vegetables

Eat more whole-grain foods, nuts, poultry, and fish

Try to limit sodium, sugary drinks, sweets, and red meat, such as beef/pork, etc.

Research has shown that you will get results within just two weeks!

Alternatively, a different form of diet known as DASH-Sodium calls for cutting down sodium to about 1,500 mg per day (which weighs about 2/3 teaspoon per day)

Generally speaking, the suggested DASH routine includes:

Daily 7-8 servings of grains

Daily 4-5 servings of vegetables

Daily 4-5 servings of fruits

Daily 2-3 servings of low-fat/ fat-free dairy products

Daily 2 or fewer servings of meat/fish/poultry

4-5 servings per week of nuts, dry beans, and seeds

Daily 2-3 servings of fats and oil

And just to give you an idea of what "Each" serving means, here are a few pointers.

The following quantities are to be considered as one serving:

½ cup of cooked rice/pasta

1 slice of bread

1 cup of raw fruit or veggies

½ cup of cooked fruit or veggies

8 ounces of milk

3 ounces of cooked meat

1 teaspoon of olive oil/ or any healthy oil

3 ounces of tofu

1 slice of bread
1 cup of raw fruit or veggies
½ cup of cooked fruit or veggies
8 ounces of milk
3 ounces of cooked meat
1 teaspoon of olive oil/ or any healthy oil
3 ounces of tofu

Some salt alternatives to know about

Letting go of salt might be a little bit difficult for people going into this diet for the first time.
To make the process a little bit easier, here are some great salt alternatives that you should know about!
Some of them are used in the recipes in our book, and you may use them if needed.

Sunflower Seeds
Sunflower seeds are fantastic salt alternatives, and they give a nice nutty and slightly sweet flavor. You may use the seeds raw or roasted.
Fresh Squeezed Lemon
Lemon is believed to be a nice hybrid between citron and bitter orange. These are packed with Vitamin C, which helps to neutralize damaging free radicals from the system.

Onion Powder
Onion powder is a dry and ground spice made out of an onion bulb for those you don't know. The powder is mainly used for seasoning in many herbs! Keep in mind that onion powder and onion salt are two different things.
We are using onion powder here. They sport a nice mix of sweet, spicy, and a bit of an earthy flavor.

Black Pepper Powder
Black pepper powder is also a salt alternative that is native to India. You may use them by grinding whole peppercorns!

Cinnamon
Cinnamon is a very well-known and savory spice that comes from the inner bark of trees. Two varieties of cinnamon include Ceylon and Chinese, and they sport a sharp, warm and sweet flavor.

Flavored Vinegar
As we call it in our book, fruit-infused vinegar or a flavored vinegar is a mixture of vinegar combined with fruits to give a nice flavor. These are excellent ingredients to add a bit of flavor to meals without salt. Experiment to find the perfect fruit blend for you.
As for the process of making the vinegar:
*   Wash your fruits and slice them well
*   Place ½ cup of your fruit in a mason jar
*   Top them up with white wine vinegar (or balsamic vinegar)
*   Allow them to sit for two weeks or so
*   Strain and use as needed

The Health Benefits of Dash Diet
Before you move forward, let me share some of the excellent health benefits you will enjoy while you are on the program.

Lower Blood Pressure

This is perhaps the main reason why the DASH diet was even invented!

Salt is believed to be very closely related to increasing blood pressure. Therefore, the purpose of the DASH diet is to closely monitor the intake of salt and reduce it to very minute levels and improve your overall blood pressure.

Aside from the salt itself, the DASH diet also helps control potassium, magnesium, and calcium, which altogether plays a significant role in lowering blood pressure!

A balanced diet also helps control cholesterol and fat levels in your system, preventing atherosclerosis, which further helps keep the arteries healthy and strain-free.

Helps Control Diabetes

Since the Dash Diet helps to eliminate empty carbohydrates and starchy food from your diet while avoiding simple sugars, a delicate balance between the glucose and insulin level of the body is created that helps prevent diabetes.

Also:

- Lowers blood pressure
- Helps to lower cholesterol levels
- Helps in weight loss
- Gives you a healthier heart
- Helps to prevent Osteoporosis
- Helps to improve kidney health
- Helps to prevent cancer
- Helps to control diabetes
- Helps to prevent depression

The pictures in the book do not represent precisely the recipe meal.

CHAPTER 2.
BREAKFASTS

MEDITERRANEAN OMELETTE

Preparation Time: 5 minutes
Cooking Time: 10 minutes
Servings: 2

INGREDIENTS
- 3 eggs, beaten
- 1 tablespoon of ricotta cheese
- 2 oz. of feta cheese, chopped
- 1 tomato, chopped
- 1 teaspoon of butter
- ½ teaspoon of salt
- 1 tablespoon of scallions, chopped

DIRECTIONS
1. Mix up the ricotta cheese and eggs. Add salt and scallions.
2. Toss the butter in the skillet and melt it.
3. Pour ½ part of the whisked egg mixture in the skillet and cook it for 5-6 minutes or until it is solid—the omelet is cooked.
4. Then transfer the omelet to the plate.
5. Make the second omelet with the remaining egg mixture.
6. Sprinkle each omelet with Feta and tomatoes. Roll them.

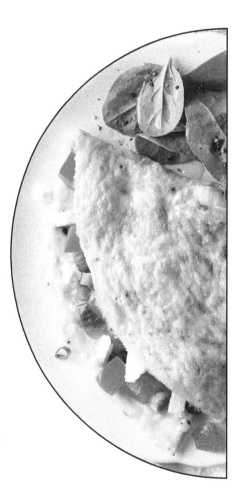

NUTRITION
- Calories: 203
- Fat: 15.2 g
- Fiber: 0.5 g
- Carbs: 3.5 g
- Protein: 13.6 g

CHICKEN FRITTERS

Preparation Time: 10 minutes
Cooking Time: 8 minutes
Servings: 2

INGREDIENTS
- 1-pound of chicken fillet, finely chopped
- 2 tablespoons of almond flour
- 1 egg, beaten
- 1 teaspoon of dried dill
- 1 teaspoon of dried oregano
- ½ teaspoon of salt
- 1 teaspoon of minced garlic
- 1 tablespoon of olive oil

DIRECTIONS
1. Put the finely chopped chicken fillet and almond flour in the mixing bowl.
2. Add beaten egg, dried dill, oregano, salt, and minced garlic. Mix it up.
3. Make the fritters.
4. Pour olive oil into the skillet and preheat it until hot.
5. Add the fritters and cook them for 4 minutes from each side over medium heat.
6. Dry the fritters with the help of the paper towel and transfer them to the serving bowl.

NUTRITION
- Calories: 284
- Fat: 14.8 g
- Fiber: 0.6 g
- Carbs: 1.4 g
- Protein: 35.1 g

EGGS IN PORTOBELLO MUSHROOM HATS

Preparation Time: 10 minutes
Cooking Time: 15 minutes
Servings: 2

INGREDIENTS
- 4 Portobello caps
- 4 quail eggs
- ½ teaspoon of dried parsley
- ¾ teaspoon of salt
- 1 teaspoon of butter, melted

DIRECTIONS
1. Brush Portobello caps with melted butter from all sides.
2. Line the tray with baking paper.
3. Put Portobello caps on the tray.
4. Beat the quail eggs into the mushroom caps and sprinkle them with salt and dried parsley.
5. Transfer the tray in the preheated to the 355 °F oven. Cook the mushrooms for 15 minutes.
6. Chill the meal a little and transfer on the serving plates.

NUTRITION
- Calories: 46
- Fat: 3.9 g
- Fiber: 0 g
- Carbs: 0.2 g
- Protein: 2.4 g

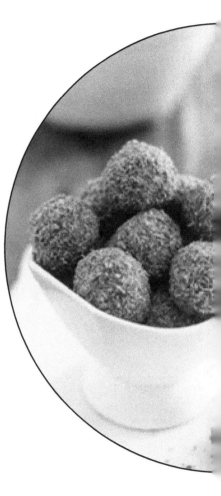

MATCHA FAT BOMBS

Preparation Time: 15 minutes
Cooking Time: 5 minutes
Servings: 2

INGREDIENTS
- ½ cup of cashew butter
- 1 cup of coconut butter
- ¼ cup of coconut cream
- 2 tablespoons of matcha green tea
- ¼ teaspoon of ground cinnamon
- ½ cup of coconut shred

DIRECTIONS
1. Put the cashew butter, coconut butter, coconut cream, ½ tablespoon of matcha green tea, and ground cinnamon in the mixing bowl.
2. Blend the mixture with the hand blender until you get a homogenous and fluffy mass.
3. In the separated bowl, combine the coconut shred and remaining matcha green tea.
4. Make the balls from the coconut butter mixture with the help of the scooper.
5. Then coat every ball in the coconut shred green mixture.
6. Transfer the meal on the plates and store them in the cold place -fridge.

NUTRITION
- Calories: 222
- Fat: 20.7 g
- Fiber: 4.1 g
- Carbs: 9.2 g
- Protein: 3.6 g

SALMON OMELET

Preparation Time: 15 minutes
Cooking Time: 5 minutes
Servings: 2

INGREDIENTS

- 3 eggs
- 1 smoked salmon
- 3 links of pork sausage
- ¼ cup of onions
- ¼ cup of provolone cheese

DIRECTIONS

1. Whisk the eggs and pour them into a skillet.
2. Follow the standard method for making an omelette.
3. Add the onions, salmon and cheese before turning the omelet over.
4. Sprinkle the omelet with cheese and serve with the sausages on the side.
5. Serve!

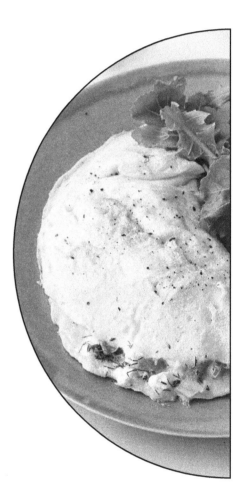

BLACK'S BANGIN' CASSEROLE

Preparation Time: 40 minutes
Cooking Time: 25-35 minutes
Servings: 2

INGREDIENTS

- 5 eggs
- 3 tablespoons of chunky tomato sauce
- 2 tablespoons of heavy cream
- 2 tablespoons of grated parmesan cheese

DIRECTIONS

1. Preheat your oven to 350 °F/175 °C.
2. Combine the eggs and cream in a bowl.
3. Mix in the tomato sauce and add the cheese.
4. Spread into a glass-baking dish and bake for 25-35 minutes.
5. Top with extra cheese.
6. Enjoy!

HASH BROWN

Preparation Time: 20 minutes
Cooking Time: 5 minutes
Servings: 2

INGREDIENTS
- 12 oz. of grated fresh cauliflower -about ½ a medium-sized head
- 4 slices of bacon, chopped
- 3 oz. of onion, chopped
- 1 tablespoon of butter, softened

DIRECTIONS
1. In a skillet, sauté the bacon and onion until brown.
2. Add in the cauliflower and stir until tender and browned.
3. Add the butter steadily as it cooks.
4. Season to taste with salt and pepper.
5. Enjoy!

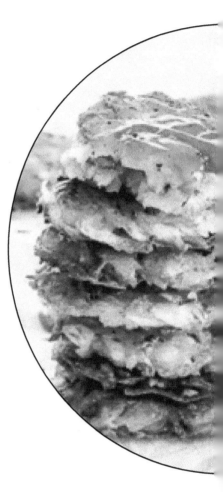

BACON CUPS

Preparation Time: 40 minutes
Cooking Time: 20 minutes
Servings: 2

INGREDIENTS

- 2 eggs
- 1 slice of tomato
- 3 slices of bacon
- 2 slices of ham
- 2 teaspoon of grated parmesan cheese

DIRECTIONS
1. Preheat your oven to 375 °F/190°C.
2. Cook the bacon for half of the directed time.
3. Slice the bacon strips in half and line 2 greased muffin tins with 3 half-strips of bacon
4. Put one slice of ham and a half portion of tomato in each muffin tin on top of the bacon
5. Crack one egg on top of the tomato in each muffin tin and sprinkle each with half a teaspoon of grated parmesan cheese.
6. Bake for 20 minutes.
7. Remove and let cool.
8. Serve!

SPINACH EGGS AND CHEESE

Preparation Time: 40 minutes
Cooking Time: 25-30 minutes
Servings: 2

INGREDIENTS
- 3 whole eggs
- 3 oz. of cottage cheese
- 3-4 oz. of chopped spinach
- ¼ cup of parmesan cheese
- ¼ cup of milk

DIRECTIONS
1. Preheat your oven to 375 °F/190 °C.
2. In a large bowl, whisk the eggs, cottage cheese, parmesan and milk.
3. Mix in the spinach.
4. Transfer to a small, greased oven dish.
5. Sprinkle the cheese on top.
6. Bake for 25-30 minutes.
7. Let it cool for 5 minutes and serve.

NUTRITION
- Calories: 346
- Fat: 11.5 g
- Fiber: 3.4 g
- Carbs: 11.5 g
- Protein: 5.6 g

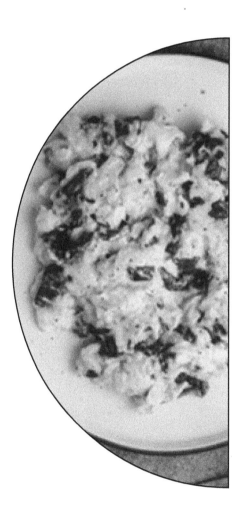

FRIED EGGS

Preparation Time: 7 minutes
Cooking Time: 5 minutes
Servings: 2

INGREDIENTS
- 2 eggs
- 3 slices of bacon

DIRECTIONS
1. Heat some oil in a deep fryer at 375 °F/190°C.
2. Fry the bacon.
3. In a small bowl, add the 2 eggs.
4. Quickly add the eggs into the center of the fryer.
5. Using two spatulas form the egg into a ball while frying.
6. Fry for 2-3 minutes until it stops bubbling.
7. Place on a paper towel and allow draining.
8. Enjoy!

NUTRITION
- Calories: 216
- Fat: 11.5 g
- Fiber: 3.4 g
- Carbs: 11.5 g
- Protein: 5.6 g

CHAPTER 3.
SEAFOOD

COCONUT MILK SAUCE OVER CRABS

Preparation Time: 10 minutes
Cooking Time: 20 minutes
Servings: 2

INGREDIENTS

- 2-pounds of crab quartered
- 1 can of coconut milk
- 1 lemongrass stalk
- 1 thumb-size ginger, sliced
- 1 onion, chopped
- 3 cloves of garlic, minced
- Pepper

DIRECTIONS

1. Place a heavy bottomed pot on medium-high fire and add all the ingredients.
2. Cover, bring to a boil, lower the fire to a simmer, and simmer for 10 minutes.
3. Serve and enjoy.

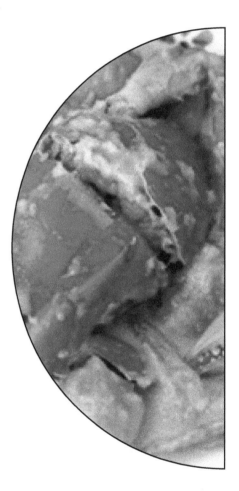

CAJUN SHRIMP BOIL

Preparation Time: 10 minutes
Cooking Time: 40 minutes
Servings: 2

INGREDIENTS

- 2 corn on the cobs, halved
- 1/2 kielbasa sausage, sliced into 2-inch pieces
- 1 cup of chicken broth, low sodium
- 1 tablespoon of old bay seasoning
- 1 teaspoon of celery seeds
- 4 garlic cloves, smashed
- 1 teaspoon of crushed red peppers
- 4 small potatoes, brushed and halved
- 1 onion, chopped
- 1-pound of shrimps
- 1 tablespoon of olive oil
- Pepper

DIRECTIONS

1. Place a heavy bottomed pot on medium-high fire and heat pot for 3 minutes.
2. Once hot, add the oil and stir around to coat the pot with oil.
3. Sauté the garlic, onion, potatoes, and sausage for 5 minutes.
4. Stir in the corn, broth, old bay, celery seeds, and red peppers. Cover and cook for 5 minutes.
5. Stir in the shrimps and cook for another 5 minutes.
6. Serve and enjoy.

SAUTÉED SAVORY SHRIMPS

Preparation Time: 10 minutes
Cooking Time: 15 minutes
Servings: 2

INGREDIENTS

- 2 pounds of shrimps, peeled and deveined
- 1 tablespoon of olive oil
- 4 cloves garlic, minced
- 2 cups of frozen sweet corn kernels
- ½ cup of chicken stock, low sodium
- 1 tablespoon of lemon juice
- Pepper
- 1 tablespoon of parsley for garnish

DIRECTIONS

1. Place a heavy bottomed pot on medium-high fire and heat pot for 3 minutes.
2. Once hot, add oil and stir around to coat the pot with oil.
3. Sauté the garlic and corn for 5 minutes.
4. Add the remaining ingredients and mix well.
5. Cover, bring to a boil, lower the fire to a simmer, and simmer for 5 minutes.
6. Serve and enjoy.

NUTRITION

- Calories: 180.6
- Carbs: 11.4 g
- Protein: 25.2 g
- Fat: 3.8 g
- Saturated Fat: 6 g
- Sodium: 111 mg

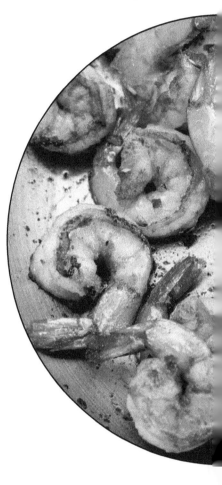

SWEET AND SPICY DOLPHIN FISH FILETS

Preparation Time: 10 minutes
Cooking Time: 25 minutes
Servings: 2

INGREDIENTS

- 2 Dolphin fish filets
- Pepper to taste
- 2 cloves of garlic, minced
- 1 thumb-size ginger, grated
- ½ lime, juiced
- 2 tablespoons honey
- 2 tablespoons sriracha
- 1 tablespoon orange juice, freshly squeezed

DIRECTIONS

1. In a heatproof dish that fits inside the saucepan, add all the ingredients. Mix well.
2. Place a large saucepan on a medium-high fire. Place a trivet inside the saucepan and fill the pan halfway with water. Cover and bring to a boil.
3. Cover the dish with foil and place on trivet.
4. Cover the pan and steam for 10 minutes. Let it rest in the pan for another 5 minutes.
5. Serve and enjoy.

NUTRITION

- Calories: 348.4
- Carbs: 22.3 g
- Protein: 38.6 g
- Fat: 2.2 g
- Saturated Fat: 5 g
- Sodium: 183 mg

STEAMED GINGER SCALLION FISH

Preparation Time: 10 minutes
Cooking Time: 30 minutes
Servings: 2

INGREDIENTS

- 3 tablespoons of soy sauce, low sodium
- 2 tablespoons of rice wine
- 1 teaspoon of minced ginger
- 1 teaspoon of garlic
- 1-pound of firm white fish

DIRECTIONS

1. In a heatproof dish that fits inside the saucepan, add all the ingredients. Mix well.
2. Place a large saucepan on a medium-high fire. Place a trivet inside the saucepan and fill the pan halfway with water. Cover and bring to a boil.
3. Cover the dish with foil and place on trivet.
4. Cover the pan and steam for 10 minutes. Let it rest in the pan for another 5 minutes.
5. Serve and enjoy.

NUTRITION

- Calories: 409.5
- Carbs: 5.5 g
- Protein: 44.9 g
- Fat: 23.1 g
- Saturated Fat: 8.3 g
- Sodium: 115 mg

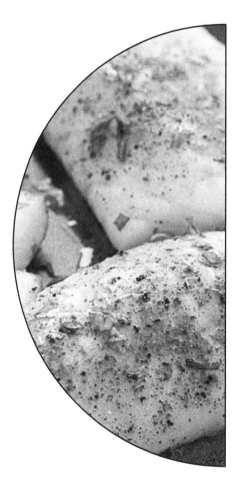

SIMPLY STEAMED ALASKAN COD

Preparation Time: 10 minutes
Cooking Time: 15 minutes
Servings: 2

INGREDIENTS

- 1-lb. of fillet wild Alaskan Cod
- 1 cup of cherry tomatoes, halved
- Salt and pepper to taste
- 1 tablespoon of balsamic vinegar
- 1 tablespoon of fresh basil chopped

DIRECTIONS

1. In a heatproof dish that fits inside the saucepan, add all the ingredients except for basil. Mix well.
2. Place a large saucepan on a medium-high fire. Place a trivet inside the saucepan and fill the pan halfway with water. Cover and bring to a boil.
3. Cover the dish with foil and place on trivet.
4. Cover the pan and steam for 10 minutes. Let it rest in the pan for another 5 minutes.
5. Serve and enjoy topped with fresh basil.

NUTRITION

- Calories: 195.2
- Carbs: 4.2 g
- Protein: 41 g
- Fat: 1.6 g
- Saturated Fat: 3 g
- Sodium: 126 mg

FISH JAMBALAYA

Preparation Time: 15 minutes
Cooking Time: 15 minutes
Servings: 2

INGREDIENTS

- 1 teaspoon of canola oil
- 1 jalapeno pepper, minced
- 1 small-sized leek, chopped
- 1/2 teaspoon of ginger garlic paste
- 1/4 teaspoon of ground cumin
- 1/4 teaspoon of ground allspice
- 1/2 teaspoon of oregano
- 1/4 teaspoon of thyme
- 1/4 teaspoon of marjoram
- 1-pound of sole fish fillets, cut into bite-sized strips
- 1 large-sized ripe tomato, pureed
- 1/2 cup of water
- 1/2 cup of clam juice
- Kosher salt, to season
- 1 bay laurel
- 5-6 black peppercorns
- 1 cup of spinach, torn into pieces

DIRECTIONS

1. Heat the oil in a Dutch oven over a moderate flame.
2. Then, sauté the pepper and leek until they have softened.
3. Now, stir in the ginger-garlic paste, cumin, allspice, oregano, thyme, and marjoram; continue stirring for 30 to 40 seconds more or until aromatic.
4. Add in the fish, tomatoes, water, clam juice, salt, bay laurel, and black peppercorns.
5. Cover and decrease the temperature to medium-low. Let it simmer for 4 to 6 minutes or until the liquid has reduced slightly.
6. Stir in the spinach and let it simmer, covered, for about 2 minutes more or until it wilts. Ladle into serving bowls and serve warm.

NUTRITION

- Calories: 232
- Total Fat: 6.7 g
- Carbs: 3.6 g
- Protein: 38.1 g

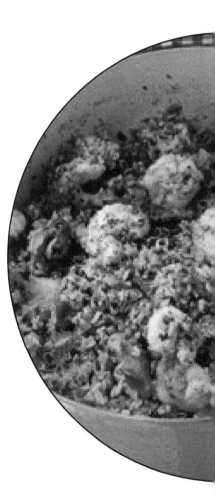

GREEK SEA BASS WITH OLIVE SAUCE

Preparation Time: 15 minutes
Cooking Time: 15 minutes
Servings: 2

INGREDIENTS

- 2 sea bass fillets
- 2 tablespoons of olive oil
- 1 garlic clove, minced
- A pinch of chili pepper
- 1 tablespoon of green olives, pitted and sliced
- 1 lemon, juiced
- Salt to taste

DIRECTIONS

1. Preheat a grill. In a small bowl, mix the half of the olive oil, chili pepper, garlic, and salt and rub onto the sea bass fillets.
2. Grill the fish on both sides for 5-6 minutes until brown.
3. In a skillet over medium heat, warm the remaining olive oil and stir in the lemon juice, olives, and some salt; cook for 3-4 minutes. Plate the fillets and pour the lemon sauce over to serve.

NUTRITION

- Calories: 267
- Total Fat: 15.6 g
- Carbs: 1.6 g
- Protein: 24 g

DINES WITH GREEN PASTA & SUN-DRIED TOMATOES

Preparation Time: 20 minutes
Cooking Time: 15 minutes
Servings: 2

INGREDIENTS

- 2 tablespoons of olive oil
- 4 cups of noodles, spiraled zucchini
- ½ pound of whole fresh sardines, gutted and cleaned
- ½ cup of sun-dried tomatoes, drained and chopped
- 1 tablespoon of dill
- 1 garlic clove, minced
- Salt and Black Pepper, to taste

DIRECTIONS

1. Preheat the oven to 350 ºF and line a baking sheet with parchment paper.
2. Arrange the sardines on the dish, drizzle with olive oil, sprinkle with salt and black pepper. Bake in the oven for 10 minutes until the skin is crispy.
3. Warm the oil in a skillet over medium heat and stir-fry the zucchini, garlic, and tomatoes for 5 minutes.
4. Adjust the seasoning.
5. Transfer the sardines to a plate and serve with the veggie pasta.

NUTRITION

- Calories: 232
- Total Fat: 6.7 g
- Carbs: 3.6 g
- Protein: 38.1 g

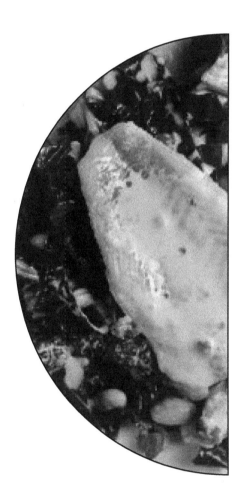

SAUCY COD WITH MUSTARD GREENS

Preparation Time: 20 minutes
Cooking Time: 15 minutes
Servings: 2

INGREDIENTS

- 1 tablespoon of olive oil
- 1 bell pepper, seeded and sliced
- 1 jalapeno pepper, seeded and sliced
- 2 stalks of green onions, sliced
- 1 stalk of green garlic, sliced
- 1/2 cup of fish broth
- 2 cod fish fillets
- 1/2 teaspoon of paprika
- Sea salt and ground black pepper, to season
- 1 cup of mustard greens, torn into bite-sized pieces

DIRECTIONS

1. Heat the olive oil in a Dutch pot over a moderate flame.
2. Now, sauté the peppers, green onions, and garlic until just tender and aromatic.
3. Add in the broth, fish fillets, paprika, salt, black pepper, and mustard greens.
4. Reduce the temperature to medium-low, cover, and let it cook for 11 to 13 minutes or until heated through.
5. Serve immediately garnished with the lemon slices if desired.

NUTRITION

- Calories: 171
- Total Fat: 7.8 g
- Carbs: 4.8 g
- Protein: 20.3 g

CHAPTER 4.
POULTRY

CILANTRO SERRANO CHICKEN SOUP

Preparation Time: 10 minutes
Cooking Time: 1 hour
Servings: 2

INGREDIENTS

- 4 chicken thighs, skin and bone-in
- 1 cup of cilantro, chopped
- 2 small Serrano peppers, chopped
- 4 and ¼ cups of low-sodium veggie stock
- 2 whole garlic cloves+ 2 garlic cloves, minced
- 2 tablespoons of olive oil
- ½ red bell pepper chopped
- ½ yellow onion, chopped
- A pinch of salt and black pepper

DIRECTIONS

1. Put the cilantro in your food processor, add Serrano peppers, 2 whole garlic cloves, and ¼ cup of stock, blend very well, and transfer to a bowl.
2. Heat a pot with the olive oil over medium-high heat, add chicken thighs, and cook for 5 minutes on each side and transfer to a bowl.
3. Return pot to medium heat, add onion, stir and cook for 5 minutes.
4. Add the bell pepper, salt, pepper, minced garlic, cilantro paste, chicken, and the rest of the stock, toss, bring to a simmer over medium heat, cook for 40 minutes, ladle into bowls and serve
5. Enjoy!

NUTRITION
- Calories: 291
- Fat: 5 g
- Fiber: 8 g
- Carbs: 10 g
- Protein: 12 g

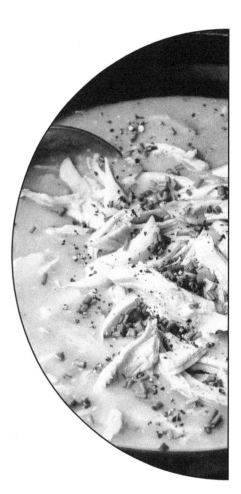

LEEK AND CHICKEN SOUP

Preparation Time: 15 minutes
Cooking Time: 1 hour and 20 minutes
Servings: 2

INGREDIENTS

- 1 lb. chicken, cut into medium pieces
- A pinch of salt and black pepper
- 3 cups of low-sodium veggie stock
- 2 leek, roughly chopped
- 1 tablespoon of olive oil
- 1/4 cup of yellow onion, chopped
- 1/8 cup of lemon juice

DIRECTIONS

1. Put the chicken in a pot, add the stock, a pinch of salt, and black pepper, stir, bring to a boil over medium heat and skim foam.
2. Add the leeks, toss and simmer for 1 hour.
3. Heat a pan with the oil over medium heat, add onion, stir and cook for 5 minutes.
4. Add this to the pot, add the lemon juice, toss, cook for 20 minutes more, ladle into bowls and serve.
5. Enjoy!

NUTRITION
- Calories: 199
- Fat: 3 g
- Fiber: 5 g
- Carbs: 6 g
- Protein: 11 g

COLLARD GREENS AND CHICKEN SOUP

Preparation Time: 10 minutes
Cooking Time: 30 minutes
Servings: 2

INGREDIENTS

- 4 cups of low-sodium chicken stock
- 1 garlic clove, minced
- 1 yellow onion, chopped
- 8 ounces of chicken breast skinless, boneless, and chopped
- 2 cups of collard greens, chopped
- A pinch of salt and black pepper
- 2 tablespoons of ginger, grated

DIRECTIONS

1. Put the stock in a pot, add garlic, chicken, and onion, stir, bring to a boil over medium heat and simmer for 20 minutes.
2. Add the collard greens, salt, pepper, and ginger, stir and cook for 10 more minutes, ladle into bowls and serve.
3. Enjoy!

NUTRITION

- Calories: 199
- Fat: 5 g
- Fiber: 5 g
- Carbs: 8 g
- Protein: 12 g

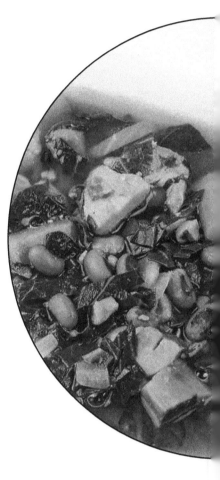

CHICKEN, SCALLIONS, AND AVOCADO SOUP

Preparation Time: 10 minutes
Cooking Time: 25 minutes
Servings: 2

INGREDIENTS

- 2 cups of chicken breast, skinless, boneless, cooked, and shredded
- 2 avocados, peeled, pitted, and chopped
- 5 cups of low-sodium veggie stock
- 1 and ½ cups scallions, chopped
- 2 garlic cloves, minced
- ½ cup of cilantro, chopped
- A pinch of salt and black pepper
- 2 teaspoons of olive oil

DIRECTIONS

1. Heat a pot with the oil over medium heat, add 1-cup of scallions and garlic, stir and cook for 5 minutes.
2. Add the stock, salt, and pepper, bring to a boil, reduce heat to low, cover and simmer for 20 minutes.
3. Divide the chicken, the rest of the scallions, and avocado in bowls, add soup, top with chopped cilantro, and serve.
4. Enjoy!

NUTRITION

- Calories: 205
- Fat: 5 g
- Fiber: 6 g
- Carbs: 14 g
- Protein: 8 g

COCONUT CHICKEN AND MUSHROOMS

Preparation Time: 10 minutes
Cooking Time: 52 minutes
Servings: 2

INGREDIENTS

- 3 tablespoons of olive oil
- 8 chicken thighs
- A pinch of salt and black pepper
- 3 garlic cloves, minced
- 8 ounces of mushrooms, halved
- 1 cup of coconut cream
- ½ teaspoon of basil, dried
- ½ teaspoon of oregano, dried
- 1 tablespoon of mustard

DIRECTIONS

1. Heat a pot with 2 tablespoons of oil over medium-high heat, add chicken, salt, and pepper, brown for 3 minutes on each side, and transfer to a plate.
2. Heat the same pot with the rest of the oil over medium heat, add mushroom and garlic, stir and cook for 6 minutes.
3. Add the salt, pepper, oregano, basil, and chicken, stir and bake in the oven at 400 °F for 30 minutes.
4. Add the cream and mustard, stir, simmer for 10 minutes more, divide everything between plates and serve.
5. Enjoy!

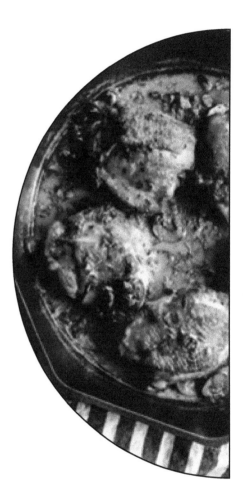

NUTRITION
- Calories: 269
- Fat: 5 g
- Fiber: 6 g
- Carbs: 13 g
- Protein: 12 g

CHICKEN CHILI

Preparation Time: 10 minutes
Cooking Time: 1 hour and 10 minutes
Servings: 2

INGREDIENTS

- 1 cup of coconut flour
- 8 lemon tea bags
- A pinch of salt and black pepper
- 4 pounds of chicken breast, skinless, boneless, and cubed
- 4 ounces of olive oil
- 4 ounces of celery, chopped
- 3 garlic cloves, minced
- 2 yellow onion, chopped
- 2 red bell pepper, chopped
- 7 ounces of Poblano pepper, chopped
- 1-quart of low-sodium stock veggie stock
- 1 teaspoon of chili powder
- ¼ cup of cilantro, chopped

DIRECTIONS

1. Dredge the chicken pieces in coconut flour.
2. Heat a pot with the oil over medium-high heat, add chicken, cook for 5 minutes on each side and transfer to a bowl.
3. Heat the pot again over medium-high heat, add onion, celery, garlic, bell pepper, and Poblano pepper, stir and cook for 2 minutes.
4. Add the stock, chili powder, salt, pepper, chicken, and tea bags, stir, bring to a simmer, reduce heat to medium-low, cover and cook for 1 hour.
5. Discard tea bags, add cilantro, stir, ladle into bowls and serve.
6. Enjoy!

NUTRITION
- Calories: 205
- Fat: 8 g
- Fiber: 3 g
- Carbs: 12 g
- Protein: 6 g

CHAPTER 5.
MEAT

PORK AND GREENS MIX

Preparation Time: 10 minutes
Cooking Time: 20 minutes
Servings: 2

INGREDIENTS

- 2 tablespoons of balsamic vinegar
- 1/3 cup of coconut aminos
- 1 tablespoon of olive oil
- 4 ounces of mixed salad greens
- 1 cup of cherry tomatoes, halved
- 4 ounces of pork stew meat, cut into strips
- 1 tablespoon of chives, chopped

DIRECTIONS

1. Heat a pan with the oil over medium heat, add the pork, aminos, vinegar, toss and cook for 15 minutes.
2. Add the salad greens and the other ingredients, toss, cook for 5 minutes more, divide between plates and serve.

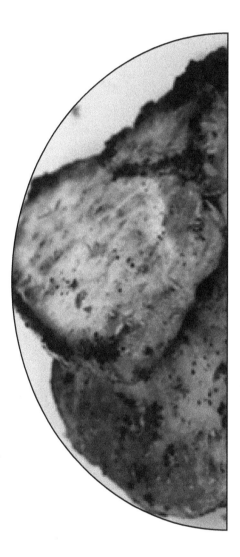

THYME PORK PAN

Preparation Time: 10 minutes
Cooking Time: 25 minutes
Servings: 2

INGREDIENTS

- 1 pound of pork butt, trimmed and cubed
- 1 tablespoon of olive oil
- 1 yellow onion, chopped
- 3 garlic cloves, minced
- 1 tablespoon of thyme, dried
- 1 cup of low-sodium chicken stock
- 2 tablespoons of low-sodium tomato paste
- 1 tablespoon of cilantro, chopped

DIRECTIONS

1. Heat a pan with the oil over medium-high heat, add the onion and the garlic, toss and cook for 5 minutes.
2. Add the meat, toss and cook for 5 more minutes.
3. Add the rest of the ingredients, toss, bring to a simmer, reduce heat to medium and cook the mix for 15 minutes more.
4. Divide the mix between plates and serve right away.

MARJORAM PORK AND ZUCCHINIS

Preparation Time: 10 minutes
Cooking Time: 30 minutes
Servings: 2

INGREDIENTS

- 2 pounds of pork loin boneless, trimmed and cubed
- 2 tablespoons of avocado oil
- ¾ cup of low-sodium veggie stock
- ½ tablespoon of garlic powder
- 1 tablespoon of marjoram, chopped
- 2 zucchinis, roughly cubed
- 1 teaspoon of sweet paprika
- Black pepper to the taste

DIRECTIONS

1. Heat a pan with the oil over medium-high heat, add the meat, garlic powder and marjoram, toss and cook for 10 minutes.
2. Add the zucchinis and the other ingredients toss, bring to a simmer, reduce heat to medium and cook the mix for 20 minutes more.
3. Divide everything between plates and serve.

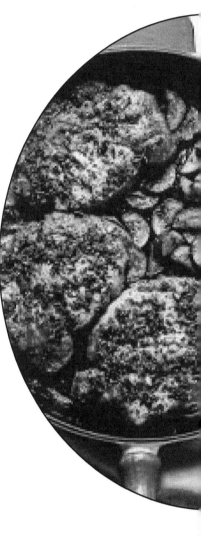

SPICED PORK

Preparation Time: 10 minutes
Cooking Time: 8 hours
Servings: 2

INGREDIENTS

- 3 tablespoons of olive oil
- 2 pounds of pork shoulder roast
- 2 teaspoons of sweet paprika
- 1 teaspoon of garlic powder
- 1 teaspoon of onion powder
- 1 teaspoon of nutmeg, ground
- 1 teaspoon of allspice, ground
- Black pepper to the taste
- 1 cup of low-sodium veggie stock

DIRECTIONS

1. In your slow cooker, combine the roast with the oil and the other ingredients, toss, put the lid on and cook on Low for 8 hours.
2. Slice the roast, divide it between plates and serve with the cooking juices drizzled on top.

COCONUT PORK AND CELERY

Preparation Time: 10 minutes
Cooking Time: 35 minutes
Servings: 2

INGREDIENTS

- 2 pounds of pork stew meat, cubed
- 2 tablespoons of olive oil
- 1 cup of low-sodium veggie stock
- 1 celery stalk, chopped
- 1 teaspoon of black peppercorns
- 2 shallots, chopped
- 1 tablespoon of chives, chopped
- 1 cup of coconut cream
- Black pepper to the taste

DIRECTIONS

1. Heat a pan with the oil over medium heat, add the shallots and the meat, toss and brown for 5 minutes.
2. Add the celery and the other ingredients. Toss. Bring to a simmer and cook over medium heat for 30 minutes more.
3. Divide everything between plates and serve right away.

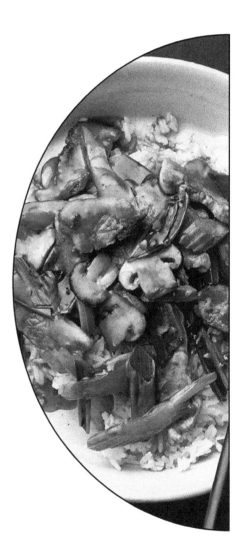

PORK AND TOMATOES MIX

Preparation Time: 10 minutes
Cooking Time: 30 minutes
Servings: 2

INGREDIENTS

- 2 garlic cloves, minced
- 2 pounds of pork stew meat, ground
- 2 cups of cherry tomatoes, halved
- 1 tablespoon of olive oil
- Black pepper to the taste
- 1 red onion, chopped
- ½ cup of low-sodium veggie stock
- 2 tablespoons of low-sodium tomato paste
- 1 tablespoon of parsley, chopped

DIRECTIONS

1. Heat a pan with the oil over medium heat; add the onion and the garlic, toss and sauté for 5 minutes.
2. Add the meat and brown it for 5 minutes more.
3. Add the rest of the ingredients, toss, bring to a simmer, cook over medium heat for 20 minutes more, divide into bowls and serve.

SAGE PORK CHOPS

Preparation Time: 10 minutes
Cooking Time: 35 minutes
Servings: 2

INGREDIENTS

- 4 pork chops
- 2 tablespoons of olive oil
- 1 teaspoon of smoked paprika
- 1 tablespoon of sage, chopped
- 2 garlic cloves, minced
- 1 tablespoon of lemon juice
- Black pepper to the taste

DIRECTIONS

1. In a baking dish, combine the pork chops with the oil and the other ingredients, toss, introduce in the oven and bake at 400 ºF for 35 minutes.
2. Divide the pork chops between plates and serve with a side salad.

NUTRITION

- Calories: 263
- Fat: 12.4 g
- Fiber: 6 g
- Carbs: 22.2 g
- Protein: 16 g

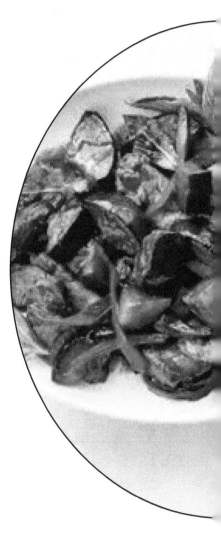

THAI PORK AND EGGPLANT

Preparation Time: 10 minutes
Cooking Time: 30 minutes
Servings: 2

INGREDIENTS

- 1 pound of pork stew meat, cubed
- 1 eggplant, cubed
- 1 tablespoon of coconut aminos
- 1 teaspoon of five-spice
- 2 garlic cloves, minced
- 2 Thai chilies, chopped
- 2 tablespoons of olive oil
- 2 tablespoons of low-sodium tomato paste
- 1 tablespoon of cilantro, chopped
- ½ cup of low-sodium veggie stock

DIRECTIONS

1. Heat a pan with the oil over medium-high heat and add the garlic, chilies, meat, and brown for 6 minutes.
2. Add the eggplant and the other ingredients bring to a simmer and cook over medium heat for 24 minutes.
3. Divide the mix between plates and serve.

NUTRITION

- Calories: 320
- Fat: 13.4 g
- Fiber: 5.2 g
- Carbs: 22.8 g
- Protein: 14 g

CHAPTER 6.
SALADS & SOUPS

PUMPKIN SOUP

Preparation Time: 10 minutes
Cooking Time: 10 minutes
Servings: 2

INGREDIENTS

- 1 chopped yellow onion
- ¾ c. of water
- 15 oz. of pumpkin puree
- 2 c. of veggie stock
- ½ teaspoon of cinnamon powder
- ¼ teaspoon of ground nutmeg
- 1 c. of fat-free milk
- Black pepper
- 1 chopped green onion

DIRECTIONS

1. Put the water in a pot, bring to a simmer over medium heat, add onion, stock, pumpkin puree, and stir.
2. Add the cinnamon, nutmeg, milk and black pepper, stir, cook for 10 minutes, ladle into bowls, sprinkle green onion on top and serve.
3. Enjoy!

NUTRITION

- Calories: 180
- Fat: 10 g
- Carbs: 22 g
- Protein: 14 g

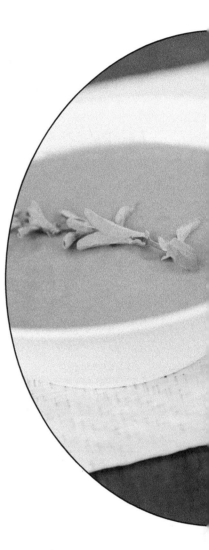

SPICY BLACK BEAN SOUP

Preparation Time: 10 minutes
Cooking Time: 1 hour, 15 minutes
Servings: 2

INGREDIENTS

- 1 lb. of black beans
- 2 chopped yellow onions
- 2 quarts low-sodium veggie stock
- 2 tablespoons of olive oil
- 6 minced garlic cloves
- 2 chopped tomatoes
- 2 chopped jalapenos
- ½ teaspoon of dried oregano
- 1 teaspoon of ground cumin
- 1 teaspoon of grated ginger
- 2 bay leaves
- 1 tablespoon of chili powder
- 3 tablespoon of balsamic vinegar
- Black pepper
- ½ c. of chopped scallions

DIRECTIONS

1. Put the stock in a pot, bring to a simmer over medium heat, add beans, cover and cook for 45 minutes.
2. Meanwhile, heat a pan with the oil over medium-high heat, add ginger, garlic and onion, stir and cook for 5 minutes.
3. Add the tomatoes, cumin, jalapeno, oregano and chili powder, stir, cook for 3 minutes more and transfer to the pot with the beans.
4. Add the bay leaves, and cook the soup for 40 minutes more while the pot is covered.
5. Add the vinegar, stir, cook the soup for 15 minutes more, discard bay leaves, blend the soup using an immersion blender, ladle into bowls and serve with scallions on top. Enjoy!

NUTRITION

- Calories: 220
- Fat: 10 g
- Carbs: 34 g
- Protein: 14 g

SHRIMP SOUP

Preparation Time: 10 minutes
Cooking Time: 25 minutes
Servings: 2

INGREDIENTS

- 8 oz. of shrimp
- 1 stalk lemongrass
- 2 grated ginger
- 6 c. of low-sodium chicken stock
- 2 chopped jalapenos
- 4 lime leaves
- 1½ c. of chopped pineapple
- 1 c. of chopped shiitake mushroom caps
- 1 chopped tomato
- ½ cubed bell pepper
- 1 teaspoon of stevia
- ¼ c. of lime juice
- 1/3 c. of chopped cilantro
- 2 sliced scallions
- 1 tbsp. fish sauce

DIRECTIONS

1. In a pot, mix the ginger with lemongrass, stock, jalapenos and lime leaves, stir, bring to a boil over medium heat, cover, cook for 15 minutes, strain liquid in a bowl and discard solids.
2. Return the soup to the pot, add pineapple, tomato, mushrooms, bell pepper, sugar and fish sauce, stir, bring to a boil over medium heat, cook for 5 minutes, add shrimp and cook for 3 more minutes.
3. Add the lime juice, cilantro and scallions, stir, ladle into soup bowls and serve.
4. Enjoy!

NUTRITION

- Calories: 190
- Fat: 8 g
- Carbs: 30 g
- Protein: 6 g

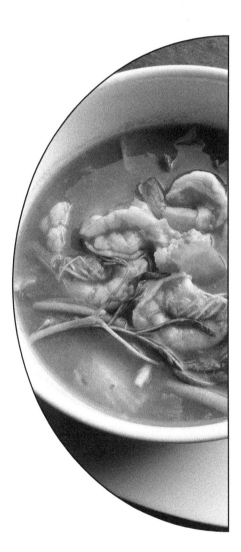

MAYO-LESS TUNA SALAD

Preparation Time: 5 minutes
Cooking Time: 5 minutes
Servings: 2

INGREDIENTS

- 5 oz. of tuna
- 1 tablespoon of extra virgin olive oil
- 1 tablespoon of red wine vinegar
- ¼ c. of chopped green onion
- 2 c. of arugula
- 1 c. of cooked pasta
- 1 tablespoon of Parmesan cheese
- Black pepper

DIRECTIONS

1. Combine all your ingredients into a medium bowl.
2. Split the mixture between two plates.
3. Serve, and enjoy.

NUTRITION

- Calories: 213.2
- Protein: 22.7 g
- Carbs: 20.3 g
- Fat: 6.2 g

CHAPTER 7.
DRESSINGS, SAUCES & SEASONING

HOT SAUCE

Preparation Time: 15 minutes
Cooking Time: 15 minutes
Servings: 2

INGREDIENTS

- 1 tablespoon of olive oil
- 1 cup of carrot, peeled and chopped
- ½ cup of yellow onion, chopped
- 5 garlic cloves, minced
- 6 habanero peppers, stemmed
- 1 tomato, chopped
- 1 tablespoon of fresh lemon zest
- ¼ cup of fresh lemon juice
- ¼ cup of balsamic vinegar
- ¼ cup of water
- Salt and ground black pepper, as required

DIRECTIONS

1. Heat the oil in a large pan over medium heat and cook the carrot, onion, and garlic for about 8-10 minutes, frequently stirring.
2. Remove the pan from heat and let it cool slightly.
3. Place the onion mixture and the remaining ingredients in a food processor and pulse until smooth.
4. Return the mixture into the same pan over medium-low heat and simmer for about 3-5 minutes, stirring occasionally.
5. Remove the pan from heat and let it cool completely.
6. You can preserve this sauce in the refrigerator by placing it into an airtight container.

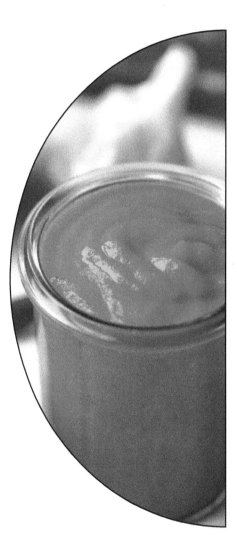

NUTRITION

- Calories: 9
- Net Carbs: 1 g
- Carbohydrates: 1.3 g
- Fiber: 0.3 g
- Protein: 0.2 g
- Fat: 0.4 g
- Sugar: 0.7 g
- Sodium: 7 mg

WORCESTERSHIRE SAUCE

Preparation Time: 5 minutes
Cooking Time: 5 minutes
Servings: 2

INGREDIENTS

- ½ cup of organic apple cider vinegar
- 2 tablespoons of low-sodium soy sauce
- 2 tablespoons of water
- ¼ teaspoon of ground mustard
- ¼ teaspoon of ground ginger
- ¼ teaspoon of garlic powder
- ¼ teaspoon of onion powder
- 1/8 teaspoon of ground cinnamon
- 1/8 teaspoon of ground black pepper

DIRECTIONS

1. Add all the ingredients to a small pan and mix well.
2. Now, place the pan over medium heat and bring it to a boil.
3. Adjust the heat to low and simmer for about 1-2 minutes.
4. Remove the pan from heat and let it cool completely.
5. You can preserve this sauce in the refrigerator by placing it into an airtight container.

NUTRITION

- Calories: 5
- Net Carbs: 0.4 g
- Carbohydrates: 0.5 g
- Fiber: 0.1 g
- Protein: 0.2 g
- Fat: 0 g
- Sugar: 0.3 g
- Sodium: 177 mg

CHAPTER 8.

SNACKS

CELERY STICKS

Preparation Time: 10 minutes
Cooking Time: 10 minutes
Servings: 2

INGREDIENTS

- 2 cups of rotisserie chicken, shredded
- 6 celery sticks cut in halves
- 3 tablespoons of hot tomato sauce
- 1/4 cup of mayonnaise
- 1/2 teaspoon of garlic powder
- Some chopped chives for serving
- Salt and black pepper to the taste

DIRECTIONS

1. In a bowl, mix chicken with salt, pepper, garlic powder, mayo, tomato sauce and stir well.
2. Arrange the celery pieces on a platter, spread chicken mix over them, sprinkle some chives, and serve.

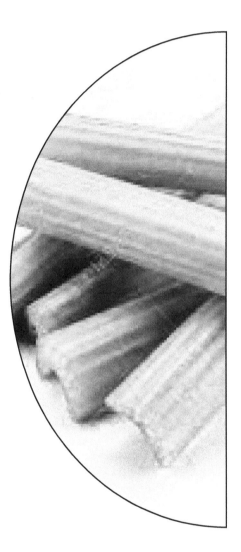

DELIGHTFUL CUCUMBER CUPS

Preparation Time: 10 minutes
Cooking Time: 10 minutes
Servings: 2

INGREDIENTS

- 2 cucumbers, peeled, cut into ¾ inch slices, and some of the seeds scooped out
- 1/2 cup of sour cream
- 2 teaspoons of lime juice
- 1 tablespoon of lime zest
- 6 ounces of smoked salmon, flaked
- 1/3 cup of cilantro, chopped.
- A pinch of cayenne pepper
- Salt and white pepper to the taste

DIRECTIONS

1. In a bowl, mix salmon with salt, pepper, cayenne, sour cream, lime juice and zest, cilantro and stir well.
2. Fill each cucumber cup with this salmon mix, arrange on a platter and serve as an appetizer.

CHAPTER 9.
DESSERTS

CREAMY DESSERT SMOOTHIE

Preparation Time: 5 minutes
Cooking Time: 10 minutes
Servings: 2

INGREDIENTS

- 175 ml cup of coconut milk
- 60 ml of sour cream
- 2 tablespoons of flaxseed meal
- 1 tablespoon of macadamia nut oil
- 20 drops of stevia
- ½ teaspoon of mango essence
- ¼ teaspoon of banana essence
- Crushed ice

DIRECTIONS

1. Start by preparing all the ingredients together, then add the flaxseed meal to some coconut milk in a bowl and let it soak up for 10 minutes.
2. Stir in the sour cream, macadamia oil, stevia, mango essence, banana essence, and mix. Add this to a blender and whisk until smooth.
3. Pour into tall glasses and add crushed ice to them.
4. Serve chilled.
5. Enjoy!

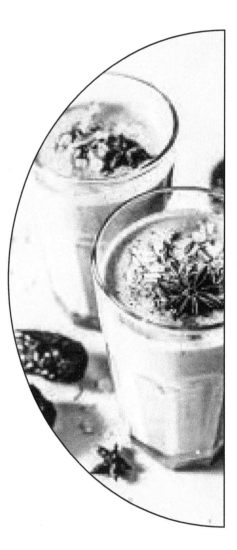

SWEET BUNS

Preparation Time: 40 minutes
Cooking Time: 30 minutes
Servings: 2

INGREDIENTS

- 1/3 cup of psyllium husks
- 1/2 cup of coconut flour
- 2 tablespoons of Swerve
- 4 eggs
- 1 teaspoon of baking powder
- 1/2 teaspoon of cinnamon
- 1/2 teaspoon of cloves; ground
- Some chocolate chips; unsweetened
- 1 cup of hot water
- A pinch of salt

DIRECTIONS

1. In a bowl, mix flour with psyllium husks, swerve, baking powder, salt, cinnamon, cloves, and chocolate chips and stir well.
2. Add water and eggs; stir well until you obtain a dough, shape 8 buns, and arrange them on a lined baking sheet.
3. Introduce in the oven at 350 ºF and bake for 30 minutes
4. Serve these buns with some almond milk, and enjoy!

CHAPTER 10.

EXTRA RECIPES

STEAK AND EGGS

Preparation Time: 25 minutes
Cooking Time: 15 minutes
Servings: 2

INGREDIENTS
- 6 eggs
- 2 tablespoons of butter
- 8 oz. of sirloin steak
- Salt and black pepper, to taste
- ½ avocado, sliced

DIRECTIONS
1. Heat the butter in a pan on medium heat and fry the eggs.
2. Season with salt and black pepper and dish out onto a plate.
3. Cook the sirloin steak in another pan until desired doneness and slice into bite-sized strips.
4. Season with salt and black pepper and dish out alongside the eggs.
5. Put the avocados with the eggs and steaks and serve.

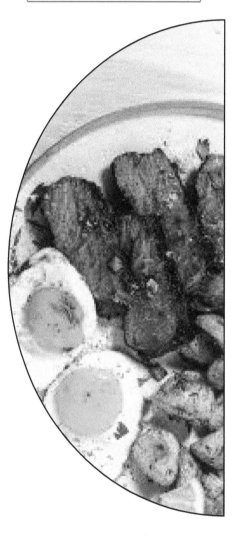

BUTTER COFFEE

Preparation Time: 20 minutes
Cooking Time: 10 minutes
Servings: 2

INGREDIENTS
- ½ cup of coconut milk
- ½ cup of water
- 2 tablespoons of coffee
- 1 tablespoon of coconut oil
- 1 tablespoon grass-fed butter

DIRECTIONS
1. Heat the water in a saucepan and add coffee.
2. Simmer for about 3 minutes and add coconut milk.
3. Simmer for another 3 minutes and allow to cool down.
4. Transfer to a blender along with coconut oil and butter.
5. Pour into a mug and serve immediately.

CALIFORNIA CHICKEN OMELET

Preparation Time: 20 minutes
Cooking Time: 15 minutes
Servings: 2

INGREDIENTS

- 2 bacon slices, cooked and chopped
- 2 eggs
- 1 oz. of deli cut chicken
- 3 tablespoons of avocado mayonnaise
- 1 Campari tomato

DIRECTIONS

1. Whisk the eggs in a bowl and pour into a nonstick pan.
2. Season with salt and black pepper and cook for about 5 minutes.
3. Add chicken, bacon, tomato and avocado mayonnaise and cover with lid.
4. Cook for 5 more minutes on medium-low heat and dish out to serve hot.

NUTRITION

- Calories: 208
- Total Fat: 15 g
- Saturated Fat: 4.5 g
- Cholesterol: 189 mg
- Sodium: 658 mg
- Total Carbohydrates: 3 g
- Dietary Fiber: 1.1 g
- Total Sugars: 0.9 g
- Protein: 15.3 g

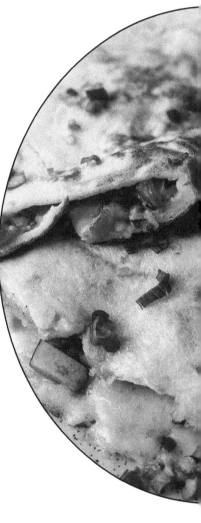

EGGS OOPSIE ROLLS

Preparation Time: 25 minutes
Cooking Time: 40 minutes
Servings: 2

INGREDIENTS

- 3 oz. of cream cheese
- 3 large eggs, separated
- 1/8 teaspoon of cream of tartar
- 1 scoop of stevia
- 1/8 teaspoon of salt

DIRECTIONS

1. Preheat the oven to 300 ºF and line a cookie sheet with parchment paper.
2. Beat the egg whites with cream of tartar until soft peaks form.
3. Mix the egg yolks, salt, stevia, and cream cheese in a bowl.
4. Combine the egg yolk and egg white mixtures and spoon them onto the cookie sheet.
5. Transfer to the oven and bake for about 40 minutes.
6. Remove from the oven and serve warm.

NUTRITION

- Calories: 171
- Total Fat: 14.9 g
- Saturated Fat: 7.8 g
- Cholesterol: 217 mg
- Sodium: 251 mg
- Total Carbohydrates: 1.2 g
- Dietary Fiber: 0 g
- Total Sugars: 0.5 g
- Protein: 8.4 g